The Ultimate Guide To CheerLeading

How To Become A Pro Cheerleader And Start To Win Everywhere

Allison Lewis

Table of Contents

Check Out My Other Books

Introduction

I want to thank you and congratulate you for purchasing the book, *"The Ultimate Guide To Cheerleading: How To Become A Pro Cheerleader And Start To Win Everywhere"*.

This book contains proven steps and strategies on how to be a pro cheerleader who can win at any cheerleading competition.

Cheerleading is one of the most exciting parts of a sports event. This is where people get to see amazing stunts and acrobatic moves that are breathtaking. Although such moves look as easy as they are spectacular, performers require years of training in order to perfect some of the most beautiful yet dangerous stunts in cheerleading contests. This book will guide you through the history of cheerleading, the exercises to improve flexibility, as well as plyometrics and other essential areas to improve on a cheerleader's body. Cheerleading may be stressful for the body, but it is also a lot of fun for those who are able to perform a stunt perfectly. If you want to be a pro cheerleader, then this book is for you.

Thanks again for purchasing this book, I hope you enjoy it!

Chapter 1: History of Cheerleading

What is the importance of history? And why should it be learned if you want to become a pro-cheerleader? Well, if you want to improve on something, you should know everything about it, including the people behind it, and the techniques they developed for future champions. Modern cheerleading is different from the original routines, but the concepts developed for the activity remain the same, and that is the history you should know about.

The first organized cheerers were all male. Their first performance dated as early as 1877 and some of the cheers yelled then are still used up to today. Cheers such as "Hurrah! Hurrah!" were yelled at different sporting events such as baseball and football. Even the athletes themselves yelled such cheers to boost the morale of their respective teams.

The first organized crowds to cheer at games were formed in 1882. The term "Cheer Leader" was first used in 1897 when three students were named as such and were assigned to cheer for their school's athletic team even during practice games. Special cheering sections in the stadium were given for them and the opposing team at the venues of the games.

The official birth of organized cheerleading was in the University of Minnesota on November 2, 1898 when the very first cheerleader directed the crowd in yelling a special cheer that is still used today. Soon after this event, a team of six male cheerleaders was organized by the university to cheer for their athletes.

In the 1940s, most men participated in the World War II. Because of this, only very few of them participate in cheerleading events, giving women the chance to dominate the sport. This is also the time when gymnastics, tumbling routines, and megaphones, were used together with the cheers. Today, studies show that 97% of all cheerleaders are female. A college level, co-ed cheerleading team consists of 50% male participants.

Many schools today assign a cheerleading team for their athletes. Modern cheerleading is closely associated with the more popular team sports such as basketball and football.

Chapter 2: The Anatomy of a Cheerleader

Modern cheerleading, with the acrobatic moves and dangerous stunts, demand a lot from the body of the participant. A cheerleader's body is expected to be in a high level of strength and flexibility, just like a gymnast or a ballet dancer. Muscular endurance is also just as important because there are stunts that have to be performed repeatedly at fast paces, which makes untrained muscles become weaker and fatigued quickly. The most important trait of a cheerleader, however, is balance. In order to perform a complicated stunt perfectly, a cheerleader should be balanced in all aspects, such as form and motion.

A strong lower body is very important for cheerleaders. Tumbling and jumping are very common sights in cheering performances. Dancing in a cheering performance requires snappy moves which also require strong lower body muscles. Many cheerleading teams have a standard in training that should be met in order for a person to be an official part of the team.

The following are a cheerleader's muscle groups that are expected to be in top conditioning:

- Upper leg muscles. This consists of the hamstrings, quadriceps, and gluteal muscles. For springy jumps and maneuvers, lower body muscle groups should be properly conditioned.

- Lower leg muscles. This consists of the gastrocnemius, Tibialis anterior muscles, and soleus. Lower leg muscles should be properly conditioned so that agile moves fast pivots, as well as standing on the ball of foot for longer periods of time can be performed easily.

- Core muscles. This consists of the abdomen, oblique muscles, and lower back muscles, the spinal erectors. These muscles need to be conditioned to be able to bend the body without experiencing pain and stress on the middle-body muscles. Many cheerleading maneuvers require bending moves and then snapping back into an upright position. Untrained middle-body muscles can be easily injured in such moves if not conditioned properly.

- Upper body muscles, the shoulder girdles. This includes the chest muscles, upper back muscles, deltoids, pectorals as well as the latissimus dorsi. Upper body muscles should be conditioned for stunts that require a participant to do a hand stand for longer periods of time. Such and similar stunts are very stressful for an untrained muscle that is why the upper body muscles should be properly conditioned for better performance.

An adequate conditioning system focusing on aspects such as strength, flexibility, endurance and balance will keep the cheerleaders performing at their best with little or no risk of injuries.

Chapter 3: Cheerleading-related Injuries

To be a professional cheerleader, you should be aware of the possible injuries you may incur while performing your stunts. Being knowledgeable about these injuries will allow you to device ways to prevent them.

Cheerleading may not be a contact sport, but a cheerleader's body is still prone to violent force and impact, especially from falls and high level maneuvers. Higher, faster, and more energetic routines increase the risks of traumatic, sometimes fatal, injuries.

As years went on, steps were developed to prevent cheerleading injuries. However, injuries are still unavoidable at some point. A cheerleader, although he is performing a stunt correctly, may stress his muscles and eventually injure himself if a correct stunt is performed repeatedly without letting that stressed body part rest. Lower and middle-body injuries are more common compared to upper body injuries, the latter, however, are usually more serious if they do happen.

The following are common cheerleading injuries that you should be knowledgeable of to be able to prevent them or to know what to do should they happen:

- Ankle injuries. Fast pivots, jumping, turning, and tumbling are some of the most common routines in a cheerleading performance. All of these moves can place too much force on one's ankles. If the ankle joint is not aligned when force is placed in it during a routine, it can lead to sprain or fracture of any bones located in that joint. A popping or grinding sensation may be felt when such injuries occur. When it happens, the affected area may not be able to handle certain weight, and swelling as well as discomfort will be felt leading to a decreased range of motion. If you suspect yourself of having fracture on your ankle, you should immediately seek medical attention. Normally, it takes 6 to 8 weeks to recover from a fracture, depending on the seriousness of the situation. Some may even require surgery in order to fully heal.

- Muscle and Tendon Strains. Dynamic cheering maneuvers that can lead to fractures may also result in muscle and tendon strains. Without proper warm up, sudden explosive maneuvers can cause tearing of muscle fibers leading to soreness, stiffness, and eventually weakness. When the muscles and tendons are not given time to rest, repetitive movements can also strain them or injure them more seriously. Cheering routines which involve exit and re-entry can help prevent muscle strains. Such exit and re-entry can let the muscles rest for a few minutes or seconds and help them recover a little before doing dynamic movements again.

- Knee dislocations and sprains. The ligaments holding the knee together will always be under stress as a person jumps, runs, and tumbles. Cheerleaders perform such moves constantly, making their knee ligaments prone to injuries. Sharp twists can tear ligaments if the lower legs do not cooperate with the twisting body. The seriousness of a knee sprain will be determined by the level of tearing that happened. If the knee is injured, the person will usually feel a lot of pain, swelling, difficulty bearing weight, decreased ranged of movement, and difficulty standing properly. Rest and less movement of the affected knee as well as ice and other medications may help in quickly recovering from a sprained knee. This recovery usually takes 4 to 6 weeks before it can be moved just like normal.

- Neck and back injuries. Somersaults gone wrong and other stunts performed without proper rehearsal usually result in bad falls. Such falls then result in neck and back injuries. Such injuries should not be taken lightly. A person who sustains neck and back injuries should remain as immobile as possible until medical personnel arrive. The spinal cord might be involved in the injury and moving the person carelessly may endanger himself further.

- Head Injuries. Just like neck and back injuries, severe trauma to the head may result to serious injury. The skull hitting a concrete floor will cause the brain to move inside, resulting into swelling and bruising. This may result to serious problems on the brain itself. Just like injuries involving the spinal cord, head injuries require medical experts' attention. A person who experienced such injury should be kept immobilized until medical personnel arrive.

Risks of injuries are always present in each cheerleading routine. Although this is a fact, such risks can be minimized by observing safety standards.

- Safety mats should be invested on for cheerleaders to be able to practice safely. A proper training environment should be given to performers so that they can practice with less risks of injury resulting from bad falls. Protective equipment should also be worn by cheerleaders.

- Proper warm-up and conditioning is a must for each person before doing strenuous activity. You can be an athlete or a cheerleader, but you won't escape the fact that you have to warm up properly before you do your sport. Sports and cheerleading demands a lot from the body, which is why you should also prepare your body for such activities.

- Flexibility is important. Flexible muscles can adapt and respond better to sharp movements and misalignments of the body during cheerleading routines and other dynamic exercises. Also, flexible muscles recover faster while moving in a wider range of motion. In short, flexibility minimizes the risks of injuries.

Chapter 4: Stretching and Other Important Exercises for Cheerleaders

Whether you like it or not, stretching is an important yet under-utilized part of a daily workout. Stretching doesn't not only improve flexibility, it also helps prevent sports related injuries such as muscle and tendon strains. Stretching also helps heal a strained muscle faster. In cheerleading, stretching is an important routine for participants to be able to perform unique stunts such as raising the legs all the way up to the head without bending the knees.

Cheerleading has a lot of stretching exercises, but there are three top stretches that should always be done by a cheerleader. Whether you are a beginner or a pro, these three stretches are essential for you to be able to do stunts without risking injury.

1. Elbow rotator stretch. While in a standing position, place your hands at the middle of your back with your elbow pointed out. Then reach your bent elbow with your other hand and gently pull it forward.

2. Knee roll over stretch while lying. Lie on your back and bend your knees. Keep your arms out to the sides and let your knees drop on one side and then to another. Keep your upper body upright and rotate only your hips as you drop your knees from one side to another.

3. High leg hamstring stretch. You need a table for this one. While standing on one foot, place your other foot on the table. Just lean forward placing your chest on your bent knee.

These are the three basic stretches that a cheerleader should always perform. There are, of course, many other stretches designed to target specific parts of the body.

The most important part of a cheerleader's stretching routine is the warm up. Without it, stretching will only tear his muscle fibers and tendons. Warm up and stretching should always be done prior to full cheerleading practice. Also, it is equally important to stretch and cool down after full practice. The only difference now is that stretches should be held longer than when the cheerleader was only warming up. This is the perfect time to increase flexibility as the muscles are already warm enough for a stretch. Each stretching exercise should be held for 15 to 20 seconds and one should go as far as feeling a little discomfort, not pain. Each stretch should be repeated 2 to 5 times.

The following are common warm up and stretching exercises for most cheerleaders:

- Shoulder rolls. Shoulders should be rolled up and around 5 times to the front then 5 times to the back.

- Hamstring stretches. The hamstrings give you flexibility as you jump. A simple yet effective stretch for this muscle is to stand up straight with feet together, then reach up and slowly bend over to reach as far down as possible, without bending your knees.

- Deltoid muscle exercise. To work out the muscles of your shoulder, take one arm and reach the opposite side of the body, without bending the elbow. Then use your other arm to pull the former arm just below the elbow. Hold the stretch for at least 5 seconds before doing the same exercise to the other arm.

- Triceps stretching exercise. These are the muscles at the back part of you upper arm. These muscles are responsible in helping you push away things. A stretching routine for this is to reach your arm up and then bend it backwards trying to reach the back part of your body, the other arm then should hold the elbow of the former arm and held for at least 5 seconds. Repeat the stretch on the other arm.

- Biceps stretching exercises. Opposite the triceps are the biceps. They are located on the front part of your upper arm. Also, their function is the opposite of the triceps. Your biceps help you pull things towards you. a stretch for these muscles is to stretch one arm in front of you, with your palms facing up. Then, using your other arm, pull the fingers of your extended arm downwards until you feel the stretch.

- Upper back and inner thigh stretches. Start in a sumo-like position with your toes facing outwards to the sides. Then, with your hands to your knees, angle one shoulder and try to reach the knee of the opposite side (without actually reaching it, you just angle until you feel the stretch). Each stretch should be held for at least 5 seconds before switching to the other side.

- Upper back stretch. This exercise is quite simple but very effective in stretching your upper back. Just stand up straight and push both arms directly in front of you while you arch your back into a "c" position. Hold the stretch for at least 5 seconds.

- Quadriceps exercise. Quadriceps is the largest muscles of your body making up the whole front part of your thigh. To stretch it, bend one leg fully backwards and hold your ankle behind you, point your knees downwards so that you won't have trouble balancing.

- Calf stretches. The calf muscles are located at the back side of the lower leg just below the back of the knee. While standing, put one foot in front of you and flex it. For balance, you can rest your arms on the supporting leg. Hold this stretch for at least 5 seconds before switching to the other side.

Other stretches for your back and legs are as follows:

- Standing leg stretches. You stand with legs half a meter apart. Bend your body all the way down until you feel the tension in your legs, then go back to the starting position and go sideways. Reach your left foot with your right hand without bending your knees. If you are more flexible, try reaching your left foot with your right elbow.

- Straddle and splitting stretches. Leg splits are good stretches for the legs, but you shouldn't force yourself to a split. Just open your legs as far as you can until you feel a slight discomfort. Then, remain in that position and stretch further by bending down forward and sideways and holding each stretch for at least 5 seconds before moving on to the next one. After all of them, slowly close your legs while massaging them. Don't close your legs quickly as it may damage your stretched muscle fibers.

- Nine Leg Stretching exercises. Sit on the floor with one leg stretched forward and the other bent inward, creating a number 9 figure. Then reach the foot of the stretched leg with your hands and try placing your head on top of your knee. Hole the stretch for at least 5 seconds before doing the same to the other side.

- Pike stretches. It's almost similar to the "nine" leg exercise only that this time your legs are together and both stretched forward. Then just bend your upper body forward as far as you can and hold such position for at least 5 seconds. Repeat at least three times, with adequate rest on each interval.

Problems on lower back flexibility are quite common among cheerleaders. Newbie cheerleaders need to work on their flexibility and they need to double the efforts on their lower back. Each cheer leading routine may require your body to bend your upper body and go back to an upright position so fast that your lower back sometimes cannot handle the tension. While new cheerleaders need stretching to improve flexibility, experienced ones need stretching to maintain them.

Cheerleaders are just like other athletes. Overworking muscles will eventually tire them out and leave them sore for days. As muscles continue to experience this without proper stretching, they will become bound and less flexible as time goes. The lower back is almost always prone to pounding each time a cheerleading stunt is performed. This is because most exercise and stunt require a lot of lower back strength and flexibility to be able to be performed perfectly. Most cheerleaders always remember stretching their legs, particularly their quadriceps, hamstrings, and other leg muscles, but they often forget to stretch their lower back muscles and gluteal muscles. Gluteal muscles and hamstrings greatly affect lower back pain and its flexibility.

The following are lower back stretches to help reduce lower back pain for athletes, cheerleaders, and everyday people alike:

- Somatic pelvic tile. This exercise is great in starting a minimal motion of the lower back without straining it too much. This is a great exercise for those experiencing significant pain on their lower back. This is also a good exercise to improve lumbar mobility. The way to do this is to lie down with knees bent. Then tilt your back upwards and remain in that position for at least 5 seconds. Repeat if necessary

- Cat stretch. You lie down on all fours. Your hands are directly positioned below your shoulders while your knees are directly positioned below your hips. You can start by arching your back going to the ceiling as you drop your head and your pelvis. Your legs and arms are to be strongly kept straight. Then return to your starting position and prepare to do the next step. Then lift your face and look at the ceiling as you keep your arms and legs strong in their position. Both sequences should be repeated at least 5 times. Remember to breathe deeply and slowly as you do this exercise. As you intensify the stretch, inhale, and as you let go of the tension, exhale.

- Seated trunk twist. This stretching exercise is performed while sitting in a chair. Trunk twists look easy, but you should be careful when doing them. Reckless twists may injure your spine. Your back should always be straight as you twist, and don't force yourself into it. you should only allow your spine to move with the twist and let it go as far as it can without forcing it. As you sit upright in a chair, place your palms on your thighs with your head directly above your shoulders. The weight of your upper body should be evenly distributed on your pelvis. As you twist to your left, place your right hand at the outside your left knee. You shouldn't exert any pressure here, placing it effortlessly and letting your spine do the twisting are enough. Allow your head freely to twist with your trunk, don't force it either. To make your twists more energized, move your eyes and look far to the side. Hold the twisting position for half a minute as you breathe slowly and deeply. Repeat the exercise on the opposite side of the body.

- Seated front bend. You can perform this exercise on a chair or on the floor, depending on your preference. However, if you lack flexibility in your lower body, you'd best be doing this while seated in a chair. For cheerleaders, on the other hand, this should be done on the floor. As you sit, place your hands on your lap while maintaining a straight body and keeping yourself relaxed. Your feet should be hip-width apart, but if you want to open it further it is fine, but you should turn your toes a little inward. Inhale, and as you exhale, lean your body forward going to your thighs. Let your hands go to either side of your feet. Remember to keep your upper body relaxed and your neck elongated. Hold this stretch for half a minute while breathing to your abdomen, and then slowly come up. This is important; you might pass out if you come up from a stretch too quickly.

Sometimes the causes of lower back pain can be hard to determine. For cheerleaders, the best way to prevent or minimize such pains is to stretch properly. Not stretching or stretching recklessly can only worsen the pain and may even affect your cheerleading performance.

Chapter 5: Stunting for Newbie Cheerleaders

Cheerleading has three basic positions that all beginners should know. As you train, you'll become an expert on at least one of them. These three positions are:

- The Base. The stunt begins with a base; this is the person on the bottom. You might think that thin small people cannot be a base, well, that is wrong. Being a base is all on the legs. As long as you have stable legs, you'd do fine. All you have to do here is to work on your leg strength. You can do squats and other plyometric exercises to improve the capacity of your legs.

- The Flyer. This refers to the person being thrown into the air. You might get excited to be a flyer, but it's not as easy as it seems. Flyers should work as hard as bases do. If you want to be the best flyer, you should remember some points:

  - Confidence. As you fly, the audience will look at you. Show them how confident you are.

- Smile. Smiling is a sign of confidence; the crowd will be amazed if you can do breathtaking stunts while you smile.

- Do not look down. Your audience is not the ground, but the people around. You should communicate with them by looking right through them.

- Be tight and firm. This will make you look more energized.

- Sell the stunt with your expressions. If the stunt is intense, show an intense expression, otherwise, it won't look real. Also, make your motions sharp to be more exciting.

- There are proper climbing techniques for flyers; practice them and use them all the time. Never improvise or make short cuts. Even if you can do them, your team mates may not be able to. And this may lead to serious injuries.

- Practice makes perfect. At home, use a mirror and check your posture for mistakes. Correct them early before going to practice to avoid delays.

- Stunting is a serious activity, laughing while doing a stunt may lead you to making mistakes. Stunts are serious maneuvers, so be serious about them.

- If you are falling, yell "DOWN", this is a general command to let your team mates know that you are falling.

- Never ever try a stunt you haven't practiced yet. Each stunt is perfected through time. If you master one stunt but perform another, you know what will happen.

To be a good flyer, you must stretch every day, practice standing on one foot for prolonged periods of time, twist on a mat, squeeze your muscles while in the air (as you jump), smile, and be confident. These are the key points to remember if you want to be a pro flyer.

- The Spotter. The spotter is the one responsible in making sure that the flyer does not fall. In many stunts, a cheerleading team has many spotters which include front and back spotters. Remember that all stunts should have a spotter. Even in the most basic stunt, someone may fall and get hurt; this is the importance of a spotter, to make sure everyone is safe.

    - Front spotter. Fronts spotters are not always needed in each stunt, but having them greatly ensures a flyer's safety.

    - Back spotter. Back spotters are usually the tallest team members. They should be able to reach the flyer's legs or feet.

An example of a stunt that distinguishes the three main positions is the Pony Mount. The base serves as the pony while the flyer sits on his back. The spotter is at the back supporting the flyer by holding onto the flyer's waist. The spotter helps the flyer get up the "pony" and dismount him.

Chapter 6: Advanced Cheerleading Stunts

There are many advanced cheerleading maneuvers, but probably the most popular one is the pyramid. The keys to a pyramid are as follows:

- The Flyer. Supposedly the lightest member of the team, the flyer is usually at the top of the pyramid.

- The Base. The member with the strongest legs is positioned at the bottom to support much weight.

- One and a half high. This pertains to the level of the pyramid. This means that the height of the pyramid is equal to one person plus half of the height another.

- Two high. Just as the one and a half high describes, two high means that the pyramid's height is that of one person standing on top of another standing person.

- Two and a half high. This pyramid's height is like that of a person standing on top of another, plus half of the height of another. Pyramids of this height are illegal in some cheerleading competitions due to the danger posed by the height of the pyramid. This type of pyramid requires additional spotters in front and back of the topmost participant.

So how do you build a pyramid? Well, a pyramid has different sections:

- Set-up. This is where all cheerleaders get into position. Flyers, bases, and spotters should first be positioned in the right place.

- Stunting and loading up. Flyers should first practice to perfect their stunts to avoid problems in loading up. Going to the top of the pyramid is a tricky maneuver, especially if the pyramid is two-and-a-half high. bases should be completely confident of their strengths to avoid the pyramid falling down and risking injury for others.

- The hit. This is where the final pose is made to "wow" the audience.

- Dismounting. Simply put, this is where the flyer jumps from the pyramid landing safely to the ground. It is important that even dismounting should be practiced slowly to avoid bad falls and injuries.

Working on a pyramid should first be done slowly. This stunt may be spectacular but it takes a lot of practice to perfect. Also, the danger posed on each member is great. Flyers may fall when outbalanced, and they may fall badly on the bases. The following are the 5 major steps in performing the pyramid:

1. Organize each side of the pyramid before putting it all together. You may ask help from spotters and catchers.

2. The second one is to load the middle bases and make sure they are strongly rooted in place.

3. Next is to load the flyers that will go to the top.

4. It would be best to rest if a member is fatigued. If one flyer comes down but the bases are still in position, try loading the flyer again. If they cannot make it, they should rest first and regain their strength; this would also help the bases not to get fatigued.

5. The one who is loaded at last should also be the one to dismount first. The flyers dismount before the bases do.

If each step is performed correctly, then you are ready to perform the pyramid easily.

Safety should always be the first priority. When a stunt is too difficult for some team members, don't pursue on doing that stunt and try other ones that seem comfortable for each member.

All cheerleading stunts are divided into three categories depending on the difficulty and risks involved. There are the basic ones, intermediate ones, and the advanced stunts. Each stunt has a degree of safety that should be followed. Advanced stunts pose a lot of threat to the participants especially the flyers. This is why each stunt should first be studied thoroughly before being tried.

Conclusion

Thank you again for purchasing this book!

I hope this book was able to help you to become a pro cheerleader who can perform anywhere given the opportunity.

The next step is to find a team to join and try everything that you have learned from this book. No sport is easy, and cheerleading is no exemption. Everything can be perfected through practice. When you have finally gained enough knowledge on the cheerleading positions, ask yourself what position best fits you, and practice well to become the top participant for that position. Each position is important and nothing is better than the other. Teamwork is the key in becoming cheerleading champions.

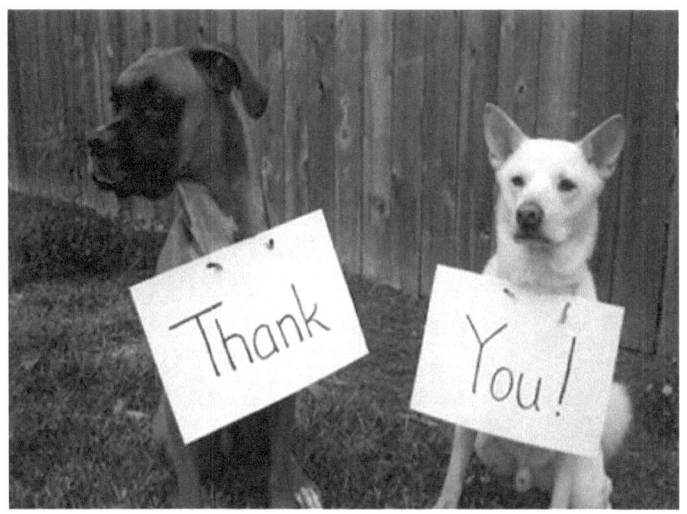

Finally, if you enjoyed this book, then I'd like to ask you for a favor, would you be kind enough to leave a review for this book on Amazon? It'd be greatly appreciated!

Thank you and good luck!

BONUS: FREE Books for You

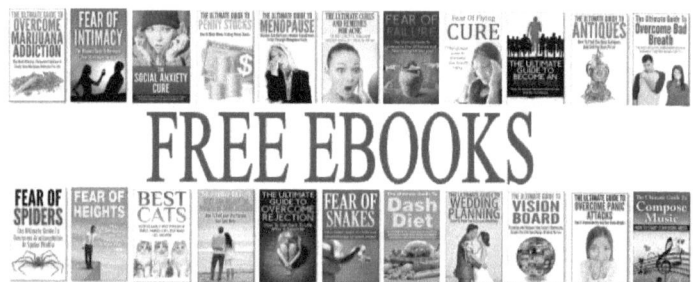

Dear reader!

If you like my books, I'd like to share more books with you FOR FREE.

When I place my book for free promotion, and the cost of the books is $ 0.00, I can send you the link for free download, and you can save up to $ 10 every time.

Simply follow the link here and let me know where to send the information about my free books. Or simply copy this link and paste it to your browser – http://bit.ly/1MD7sXu

Check Out My Other Books

Below you'll find some of my other popular books that are popular on Amazon and Kindle as well. Simply click on the links below to check them out. Alternatively, you can visit my author page on Amazon to see other work done by me. If the links do not work, for whatever reason, you can simply search for these titles on the Amazon website to find them.

1) The Ultimate Guide To Become An Alpha Female - How To Attract Men, Win In Life And Be Confident

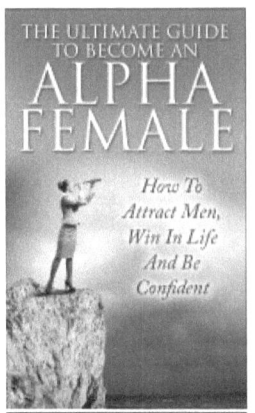

Click here to check out 'The Ultimate Guide To Become An Alpha Female - How To Attract Men, Win In Life And Be Confident ' book.

Or go to: http://amzn.to/1NFrQHv

2) How to Lose Thigh Fat - The Most Effective and Simple Solutions to Trim your Thighs

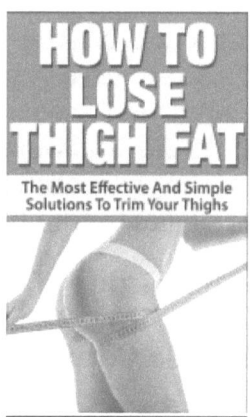

Click here to check out 'How to Lose Thigh Fat - The Most Effective and Simple Solutions to Trim your Thighs ' book.

Or go to: http://amzn.to/1Nea3Nd

Thanks You!

Allison Lewis